Praise for *You'll Know*

"These strikingly vivid portraits give the
while capturing the relentless brutality of
military history, but also to an entire nation that is grateful for the incomparable contributions of
men and women in nursing. These stories show us that no matter the era of the war and no matter
how medically prepared we are, the art and heart of nursing ultimately make the difference—nurses
who devote caring, respect, team sense, and esprit de corps to their cause."

–Diane Carlson Evans, RN
44th Medical Battalion, Vietnam, 1968-69
Army Nurse Corps, 1966-72

"I laughed; I cried; I remembered. These pages are a fitting tribute to the incredible accomplish-
ments of today's military nurses. The short vignettes are rich in accounts of daunting challenges,
unforgettable patients, and inevitable occasions of sadness that come when you care deeply about
those you serve. Yet there are also stories of the humor, camaraderie, and pride that sustain the
spirit through the toughest times. This book will spark memories and, I hope, inspire many to join
the ranks of military nurses."

–Barbara C. Brannon, Major General, USAF (Ret.)
Assistant Air Force Surgeon General for Nursing, 1999-2005

"Until now, only the military nurse and the warriors they cared for knew. This collection captures
the heart and soul of military nursing, previously an enigma to those on the outside looking in."

–Cindy Gurney, Colonel (Ret.)
U.S. Army Nurse Corps Historian

"The pride, commitment, joy, and remarkable expertise of nurses serving in the military shine through on every page of this book. The images, anecdotes, and reflections tell a story of courage, compassion, and endurance that will bring you to tears and inspire awe and gratitude. This is a powerful tribute to these often unsung heroes of the military who go above and beyond the call of duty, often in the midst of danger, to serve those in need during war and disaster."

–*Judith S. Mitiguy, RN, MS*
Former Editor-in-Chief, Gannett Healthcare Group
Commissioned Officer and Registered Nurse, U.S. Navy, 1965-68

"This book is a must-read, particularly for anyone thinking of becoming a military nurse or for military nurses who haven't served in a combat environment. More importantly, it is a must-read for all who care about our soldiers, the medical treatment they receive, their courage, and the commitment of the medical teams. To read this book and look at the pictures, and not have a tear come to the eye, seem impossible. It leaves me touched and prouder than ever of those who serve."

–*Wilma L. Vaught, Brigadier General, USAF (Ret.)*
President, Women in Military Service for America Memorial Foundation

"This book sets a precedent for military nurses finding their way into the pantheon of American history."

–*Army Lt. Col. Brad West, MSN, CRNA*
Veteran, Iraq and Afghanistan wars

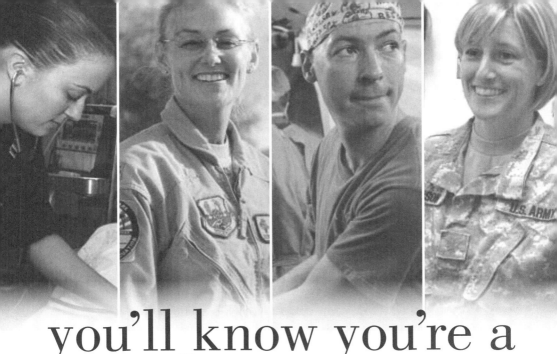

you'll know you're a
military nurse
when...

Sigma Theta Tau International
Honor Society of Nursing®

Sigma Theta Tau International

Copyright © 2011 by Sigma Theta Tau International

Sigma Theta Tau International
550 West North Street
Indianapolis, IN 46202

To order additional books, buy in bulk, or order for corporate use, contact Nursing Knowledge International at 888.NKI.4YOU (888.654.4968/US and Canada) or +1.317.634.8171 (outside US and Canada).

To request a review copy for course adoption, e-mail solutions@nursingknowledge.org or call 888.NKI.4YOU (888.654.4968/US and Canada) or +1.317.917.4983 (outside US and Canada).

To request author information, or for speaker or other media requests, contact Rachael McLaughlin of the Honor Society of Nursing, Sigma Theta Tau International at 888.634.7575 (US and Canada) or +1.317.634.8171 (outside US and Canada).

ISBN-13: 978-1-930538-96-2

Publisher: Renee Wilmeth
Principal Book Editor: Carla Hall
Acquisitions Editor: Janet Boivin, RN
Development Editors: Jane Palmer, Carla Hall
Editorial Coordinator: Paula Jeffers
Cover Designer: Rebecca Batchelor
Interior Design and Page Composition: Rebecca Batchelor

Printed in the United States of America

Printing and binding by Edwards Brothers, Inc.

First Printing, 2010

All stories for this book were collected from the *You'll Know You're a Military Nurse When* . . . website at www.militarynursebook.com. The publisher wishes to express gratitude for all who left their stories for the world community of nurses to share. The site remains open for new contributions from military nurses who have not yet had the opportunity to share his or her story.

Table of Contents

Acknowledgements. vi

Foreword vii

Introduction. ix

On the Move 3

Uniforms that Pack More
   than a Stethoscope 11

Trauma 17

Honor and Dignity 27

Band of Nurses 39

Proud to Serve. 43

Multitaskers 50

Real Life on the Front Lines 61

Rewards of the Job 67

Index of Authors. 82

Acknowledgements

The editors of Sigma Theta Tau International wish to acknowledge the following people and organizations for their assistance in producing this book: Ada Sue Hinshaw, dean, and Sharon Willis from the Uniformed Services University of the Health Sciences for their hard work in organizing a cover photo shoot for us (unfortunately, that cover could not be used); Margaret Tippy, media relations officer, U.S. Army Medical Command; Harry Sarles, public affairs officer for the Command and General Staff College, Ft. Leavenworth, Texas; Women in Military Service for America Memorial Foundation; retired Col. Jeri Graham from the Army Nurse Corps Association; and Cindy Gurney from the Vietnam Women's Memorial Foundation.

Foreword

I am honored for the opportunity to introduce you to some of my military nursing colleagues—men and women from the Army, Air Force, and Navy who share their thoughts about military nursing. I was fortunate to spend 32 years on active duty as an Army nurse and would join them again in an instant if it were possible.

I am often asked why I became an Army nurse. It was because of my father's concern for service members. He cherished the kindness of strangers who invited him into their homes for meals while he served in World War II, so he always invited soldiers to our home. One of those young men became a "big brother" to me. He was injured in an explosion in Vietnam and lost a leg. The Army health care team kept him alive and brought him home to me. I knew then that the only type of nursing I wanted to do was Army nursing. I wanted to make sure that someone else's big brother—or father, mother, son, daughter, or sister—came home alive to loved ones. It is what motivated me every day of my career, regardless of the frustrations or challenges.

You'll Know You're a Military Nurse When… focuses on our care of servicemen and servicewomen during combat. As nurses, we truly understand the pain and suffering from war. The primary reason our military has nurses is to provide care during war and conflicts, but that is not all we do. However, many military nurses say that it is the most rewarding nursing they do in their entire lives.

When we are not serving those in harm's way, we nurse in a variety of environments—clinics, community hospitals, and tertiary medical centers. Military nurses are the best educated in the nation—about 80% have master's degrees, and those who seek a doctoral education get one.

I believe that military nursing is an affair of the heart. Once you meet the military patients and those who love them, something magical happens. They become the reason that you cope with the myriad of experiences that accompany military life. Your love and dedication to those patients overcome the little irritants that occur in life, and you go to work with a passion that few others understand.

The men and women who contribute their voices to *You'll Know You're a Military Nurse When…* are leaders who will raise nursing in the United States to higher standards and take nursing into new places. They understand the importance of teamwork, communication, patient safety, and excellence in professional nursing. They thrive on continual learning and professional growth, and they do not settle for the status quo.

I am certain you will enjoy these thoughts from America's military nursing heroes!

–Gale S. Pollock
Major General (Ret.)
22nd Chief, Army Nurse Corps

Introduction

I am not a military nurse, but I have been writing about Air Force, Army, Navy, Reserve, and National Guard nurses for many years. No matter how many military nurses I interview or how many of their stories I write, I believe I will never fully understand what it is like to be a member of such a select, self-sacrificing group.

Florence Nightingale, the most famous of all nurses, gained her fame and proved the value of good nursing care during the Crimean War. Clara Barton, America's best known nurse and founder of the American Red Cross, earned her reputation on the bloody battlefields of the American Civil War.

The work of contract nurses during the Spanish-American War at the end of the 19th century proved to the Army that it needed a professional nursing corps, which it established in 1901. The Navy formed its own corps in 1908. When the Air Force was founded in 1947, the Air Force Nurse Corps followed a year later.

In each successive war, military nurses have helped increase the number of wounded service members who survive their injuries, just as Nightingale and Barton did. To do so, they often put their own lives at risk as military nurses, physicians, and medics are moved closer to the front lines. In Iraq and Afghanistan, technology, combined with the ability to rapidly implement lessons learned from the battlefield, have helped achieve a survival rate of about 95%.

Military nurses today work in small teams of highly specialized and trained medical personnel. Air Force nurses are members of critical care air transport teams that are literally ICUs in the sky; Navy nurses accompany Marines into the fiercest of fighting as members of shock trauma platoons, and Army operating room nurses and CRNAs (certified registered nurse anesthetists) help surgeons operate far forward on the battlefield. Military nurses also conduct research in Iraq and Afghanistan. No lesson learned is wasted.

As are most RNs, military nurses can be reluctant to talk about their contributions to saving the lives of service members or comforting the men and women who do not make it home. For that reason, the Honor Society of Nursing, Sigma Theta Tau International decided to encourage military nurses to tell their own stories. And so, we launched a military nurse web page— www.militarynursebook.org—where nurses could complete the statement "You'll know you're a military nurse when…" for possible publication in a book.

This is that book. It is a compelling collection of the quotes, comments, anecdotes, and thoughts military nurses wrote on militarynursebook.org that best illustrate to us what it means to be a military nurse. We hope that this little book makes military nurses proud and that it helps others understand the service contributions of uniformed nurses.

–Janet Boivin, RN
Book Acquisitions Editor
Honor Society of Nursing, Sigma Theta Tau International

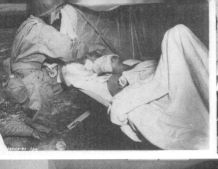
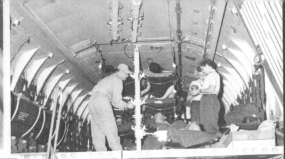
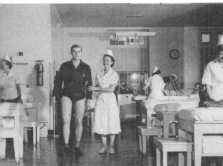
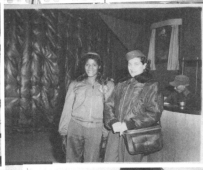
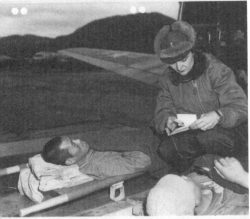
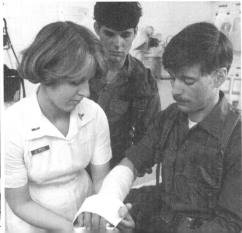

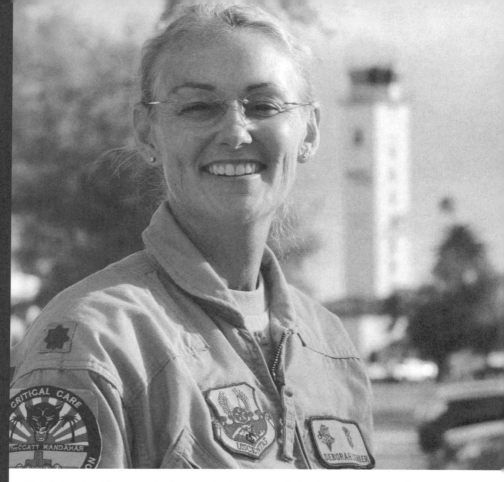

Maj. Deborah Lehker served a 6-month deployment to Afghanistan as a nurse with a critical care transportation team. (U.S. Air Force photo/Tech. Sgt. Carolyn Erfe)

on the move

"…You are flying in the back of a Marine helicopter at 500 feet with two ventilated patients and somehow, between worrying about your patients and your own life, you find time to wonder what the Joint Commission would think of this activity and whether the Environment of Care Committee would approve of it."

–George Dyer, Navy, TQ Surgical Company, Camp Al Taqaddum, Iraq

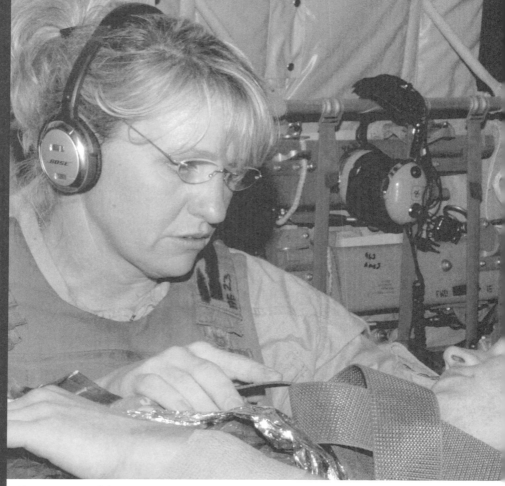

"…You are asked what part of the hospital you work in and you say, 'I don't.' After the puzzled look, you tell them that you are a nurse on airplanes, and the confusion grows even further. I explain that I am an Air Force flight nurse, and my job is aeromedical transport. I explain how I have played a vital role in making the wars in Iraq and Afghanistan the most survivable wars in history. I say if you are injured and make it to one of the U.S. military hospitals in Balad, Mosul, Kandahar, or Bagram, you have a 98% chance of surviving— the highest the nation has ever achieved. Many also find it amazing that a critically ill patient will be in a state-of-the-art ICU in the States within 72 hours of injury in Iraq or Afghanistan. The people I serve with make this happen. Being a flight nurse is challenging and not so high-tech. While I write this, I am in Iraq with average temperatures of 120 degrees. I sweat setting up the aircraft with our 400 pounds of gear. My mission may be routine, priority, or urgent, but it does not matter. My goal is to give the best care possible."

–Delisa Showers
Air Force, 459th Aeromedical Evacuation Squadron
Balad, Iraq

"…You find yourself saluting a UH-60 MEDEVAC (medical evacuation) helicopter as it takes off in a cloud of dust, highlighted by green lights and carrying away the soldiers that you could not save on your trauma bed in Baghdad that day."

–Amber Birkle, Army, Blanchfield Army Community Hospital and 10th Combat Support Hospital, Bassett Army Community Hospital, Baghdad, Iraq

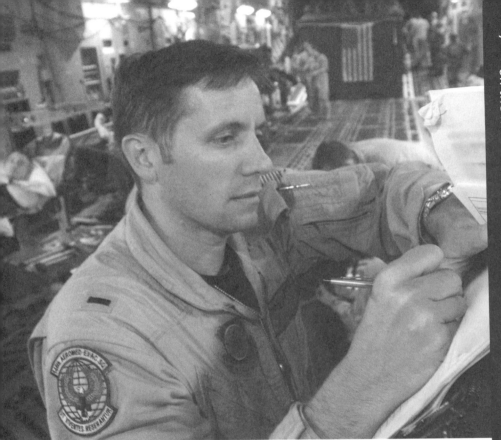

1st Lt. John Rinaldo annotates a patient's records after completing an aeromedical evacuation mission on a C-17 Globemaster III. Rinaldo is a flight nurse serving temporary duty with the 791st Expeditionary Aeromedical Evacuation Squadron at Ramstein Air Base, Germany. (U.S. Air Force photo/Master Sgt. John E. Lasky)

…You are caring for 30-plus wounded troops in the back of a dark, cold, and noisy aircraft cargo bay while wearing Kevlar body armor, helmet, and other combat gear. Caring for wounded troops in the back of a cargo plane is one of the biggest challenges for an Air Force flight nurse. The environment is in constant flux. The temperature will be 110 degrees when bringing the wounded onboard and then 60 degrees when the aircraft reaches altitude. The aircraft engine is so loud that you cannot hear lung and heart sounds or monitor alarms; yelling is the only form of communication. Lighting is extremely limited, since the mission is flown at night and low lights are used to prevent enemy fire.

In addition, the vibration from the aircraft makes ECG monitoring difficult and pain management for troops with orthopedic injuries difficult at best. Changes in altitude also add significant stressors to the wounded troops. For example, barometric changes increase a pneumothorax; decreased oxygen concentration causes havoc for the already hypoxic patient. Then there is dehydration and fatigue.

These stressors of flight affect not only the wounded but also those caring for them. Our days are long, from 12 to 24 hours at a time; the planes are packed with 30 to 60 wounded; the environment is hot and noisy; and the enemy likes to shoot at the plane. At the end of the day, when you are walking off the plane tired, dirty, and ready for bed, there is always a smile for a mission well done— because it is still the best job in the world.

–Diane Doty, Air Force, 445th Air Evacuation Squadron, Balad Air Base, Iraq

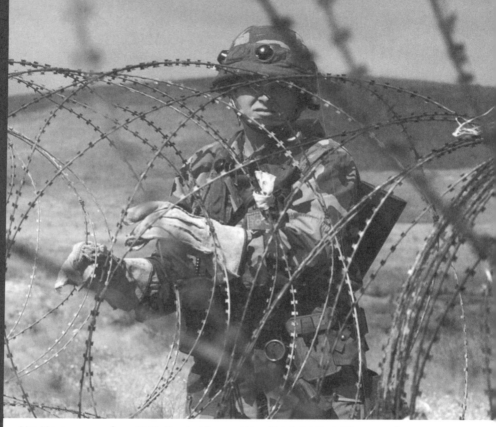

Lisa Mayer, a nurse from 114th Combat Support Hospital, Saint Paul, Minnesota, forms a border with concertina wire during Operation GOLDEN MEDIC. Reserve forces from all over the nation participated in the multi-unit, medical field exercise held at Parks Reserve Forces Training Area, Dublin, California, in which the Army transported simulated casualties from the front line through various staging areas to a main tent. (U.S. Air Force photo/Tech. Sgt. Robert A. Whitehead)

uniforms that
pack more than
a stethoscope

you'll know you're a military nurse when …

"…You can crawl under barbed wire in the morning and don your dress uniform for a ball that evening."

–Lois Borsay, Army, Landstuhl Regional Medical Center, Landstuhl, Germany

"…Something changes internally for you when you put on your uniform. The flag is the symbol of the country that we proudly represent. The uniform represents which branch of the service we have chosen to serve. But the nursing shield is unnoticeable to the eye, because it is held deep within our hearts."

–Lillian Cardona, Army, 212th Mobile Army Surgical Hospital, Germany

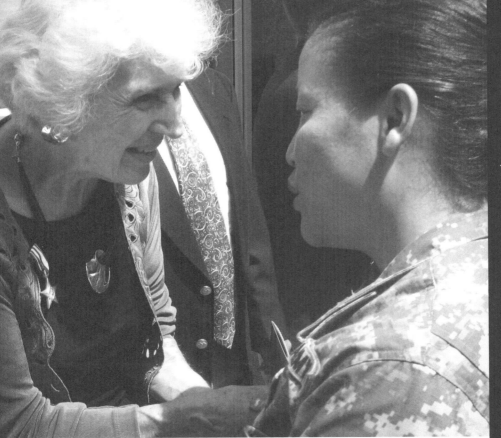

Mary Jane Bolles Reed talks with Capt. Rachel Park, the assistant head nurse for the surgical intensive care unit at Walter Reed Army Medical Center, after accepting the Silver Star on behalf of her late mother, Linnie Leckrone, an Army nurse who was one of the first females authorized to wear the Silver Star. (Photo: Fred W. Baker III)

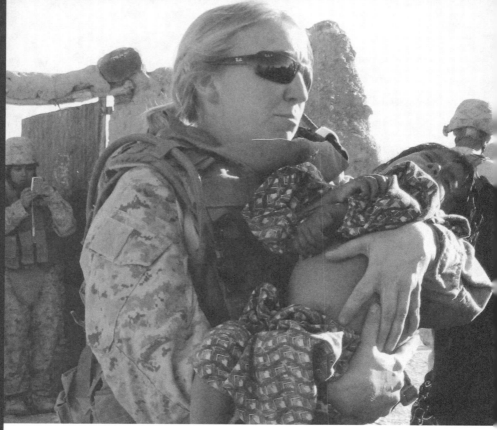

Lt. Amy Zaycek, the severe trauma platoon nurse with the Female Corpsman Team (FCT), holds an Afghan child during a patrol in the area of Now Zad, Afghanistan. The FCT returned to Now Zad to assist members of the Female Engagement Team, Marine Expeditionary Brigade-Afghanistan, with their effort to further the process of treating, educating, and engaging the women of Now Zad. (1st Marine Division Public Affairs/Cpl. Zachary Nola)

"…You wake up and don your U.S. Army combat uniform complete with boots and dog tags; accessorize it with a stethoscope, trauma shears, and a penlight; and feel more pride in that uniform than in hospital scrubs."

–Amber Birkle, Army, Blanchfield Army Community Hospital and 10th Combat Support Hospital, Bassett Army Community Hospital, Baghdad, Iraq

"…Instead of packing a lunch every day, you're packing a 9mm pistol to take with you to work."

–Michelle Ortiz, Navy, Djibouti City, Djibouti, Africa

"…You can work a double shift, wearing your standard-issue government combat boots, and still care far more about your 'battle buddies' (who just so happen to be your patients) than your own aching feet. Hooah!!"

–Cynthia Kinsey, Army, Ft. Knox, Kentucky

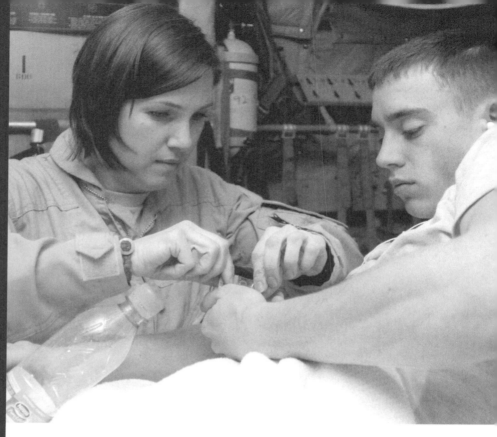

Capt. Susan McCormick gives medicine to Airman 1st Class Brent Noah during an aeromedical evacuation flight to Bagram Airfield, Afghanistan. Noah, assigned to the 376th Expeditionary Aircraft Maintenance Squadron at Manas Air Base, Kyrgyzstan, dislocated his hip and was being flown to Bagram Airfield for treatment. McCormick is a flight nurse with the 455th Expeditionary Aeromedical Evacuation Flight at Bagram. (U.S. Air Force photo/Senior Airman Erik Cardenas)

trauma

"…You say, 'War is hell,' and you know it is true because you lived through it. You say nothing could have prepared you for this—no textbook, no clinical rotation, no virtual lab—because no trauma center has ever experienced the types of horrific injuries that you've seen and taken care of."

–*Mary Carlisle, Air Force, 332nd Expeditionary Medical Group, Balad, Iraq*

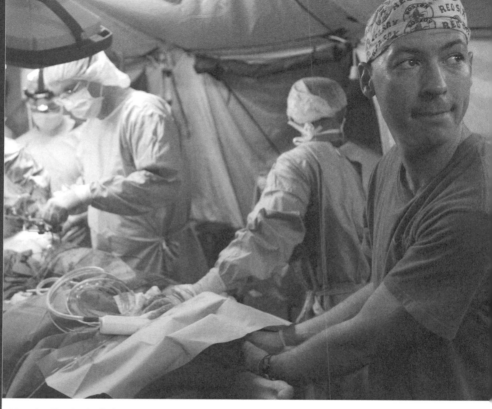

Navy Lt. Charles L. Cather, an operating room nurse assigned to the Surgical/Shock Trauma Platoon (SSTP) at Camp Taqaddum, Iraq, pulls on a patient's leg during surgery to prevent the leg muscle from retracting during surgery. The SSTP, part of the 1st Force Service Support Group, was one of three major immediate surgical and trauma care teams assigned to Marine forces operating in Iraq. In the first 6 days of combat operations in Fallujah, the 63 surgeons, nurses, corpsmen, and other personnel of the SSTP treated 157 patients and operated on 73 of them. (U.S. Marine Corps photo/Staff Sgt. Jim Goodwin)

"…You learn that your next patient for surgery is from OEF (Operation Enduring Freedom), and you are thrilled to see he has all his limbs. The scariest part of the continued war operations is the IED (improvised explosive device) blast injuries that are changing the way young men and women will forever live their lives. To see wounded service members— fresh off the plane from the Army hospital in Landstuhl, Germany, looking like they are just one breath away from dying—and eventually watch some of them walk out of the hospital gives me trust in the miracles wrought by trauma teams and God.

"To call and give a mother an update on her son during surgery, and the first question out of her mouth is, 'Does he have five fingers?' truly humbled me. I remembered asking that same question each time my own children were born. However, this mother was hoping we could save the only five fingers her son had left. I often feel I am not worthy to care for these heroes, but I am honored to be involved in their lives."

–Tamara Braghieri, Navy, National Naval Medical Center, Bethesda, MD; Naval Medical Center Portsmouth, VA; Naval Hospital Jacksonville, FL; Naval Hospital Oak Harbor, WA

…On the first day you completely take over for another unit, there is a MASCAL (mass casualty), and it turns out to be your first MASCAL, your first DOA (dead on arrival), and your first MEDEVAC. We had arrived at the Abu Ghraib prison to relieve an Army Reserve unit. A call came in that a Marine Humvee was hit by an IED. One Marine was DOA, another had only scratches, and a third came in all torn up and had gray matter showing. I remember he was bleeding everywhere. After the trauma assessment, they rushed him to the OR to stop the bleeding and do damage repair.

My chief nurse told me I was going to fly him to Balad. I took liters and liters of fluid and blood, as well as medications. All I remember is that this Marine was bandaged up, and I didn't know what he looked like; he was just a name. In flight, the ventilator cut off. My flight medic was bagging him with the ambu bag as I was pushing fluids in him. His blood pressure was waxing and waning, and I couldn't get a pulse oximetry reading anywhere on him. I realized this was someone's son, someone's husband, someone's brother. My prayer was that he stay alive at least until his family said goodbye. I told him, 'Don't you dare leave me!' The Black Hawk helicopter was flying exceptionally low because of the poor visibility, which made the bird a greater target. But I had no time to worry about that. We arrived at Balad Air Base after a shaky flight, and I handed the Marine off to the Balad crew. My flight medic asked if that was my first MEDEVAC, and I replied, 'Yes.' He told me that to survive, I had to shake it off. The Marine had a pulse and was alive when I dropped him off, and that was it.

I found out later the Marine had made it to National Naval Medical Center in Bethesda, Maryland. I wrote a note to the family, explaining how he was our unit's hero and what the hospital did to save him. A day later, my inbox was flooded with e-mails from his family as well as his church people. They were so grateful for our unit, and they said my letter was an answered prayer to them. This experience was the rock that I leaned on when things got tough throughout that year. To this day, I keep in contact with his family. He went through cranioplasty and is almost completely functional. The family and I plan to meet one day."

–Rachel Park, Army, 21st Combat Support Hospital, Baghdad, Iraq

"…At age 28 you are the only nurse, and the only one with critical care experience, for more than 3,000 soldiers and Marines in the hostile city of Ar Ramadi in 2003-04, and you chose to be there!"

–Jodelle Schroeder, Army, 101st Forward Support Battalion, 1st Brigade, 1st Infantry Division (mechanized), Ar Ramadi, Iraq

"…You have a soldier who just returned from war with devastating injuries and is in terrible pain, and he apologizes for cursing at an officer. You watch a dying soldier get his Purple Heart while his mother smiles proudly. Then he turns to you and says, 'It hurts too bad to get this medal.' You have to tell a 20-year-old infantryman that he no longer has legs, because since his injury, he has been too sedated to know that he was blown in half. You do your 12-hour shift, and then take time to check on the soldiers who have actually made it out of your ICU to the ward—just to see how they are doing—and they are so happy to see you."

–Christina Cooper, Army, C Company, Walter Reed Army Medical Center

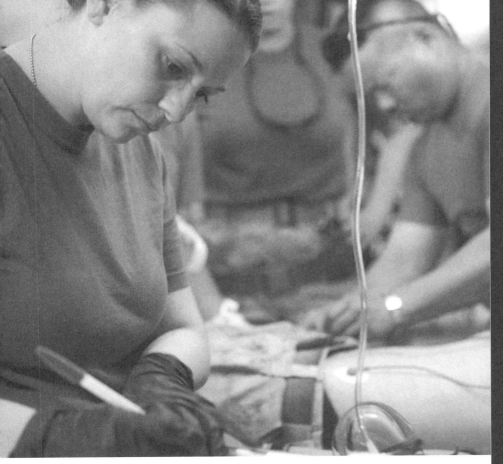

Registered nurse Lt. j.g. Phyllis Dykes records doctors' notes while staff members of the Combat Logistics Battalion 8 Surgical Support Team examine a new patient. (Gunnery Sgt. Chris W. Cox)

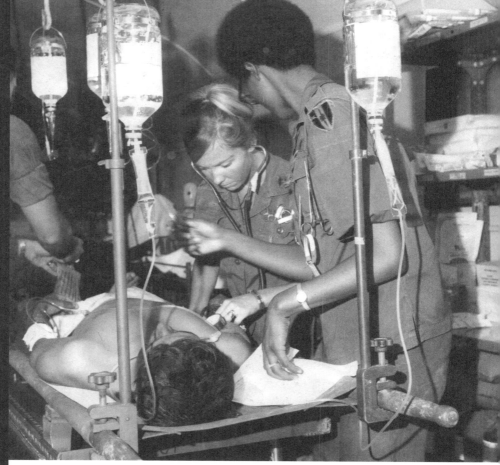

Army nurses, 93rd Evacuation Hospital, Long Binh, Vietnam, 1968. (B.J. [Greenway] Rasmussen Collection, Women In Military Service For America Memorial Foundation, Inc.)

"…You spend the rest of your life worrying and praying for patients whose names you don't even remember. Two days before leaving Vietnam, one young man, Bobby, started to wake up from his surgery. He opened one eye and asked me, 'How many?' I asked what he meant, and he replied, 'How many of my legs are gone?' I had to tell this 19-year-old that he had lost both legs. I spent every free moment I could with him until I had to leave the hospital to catch my freedom bird. I was only 21, married, and going home with my husband, who had no physical injuries. I knew that I was sending Bobby home with many physical and psychological scars. Over the past 40 years, I have wondered what happened to Bobby and if he had a good life. He is in my thoughts and prayers. I carry Bobby and many of my nameless patients with me."

–Paula Quindlen, Army, 27th Surgical, Chu Lai, South Vietnam

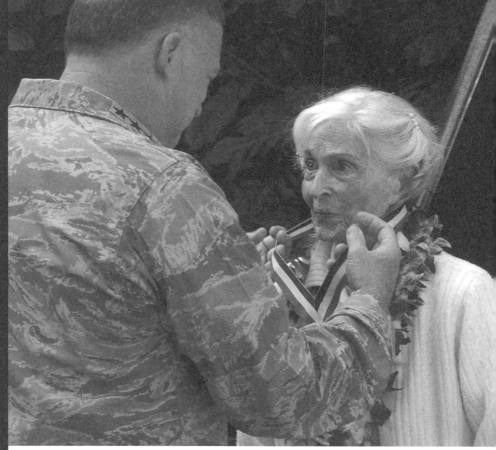

Gen. Gary North presents a medallion to Doris Avery, a member of the "Greatest Generation," to honor her efforts in World War II, at Joint Base Pearl Harbor Hickam, Hawaii. North, the Pacific Air Forces commander, presented the Noncommissioned Officers' Association World War II Veterans Medallion to Avery for her heroic efforts. (U.S. Air Force photo/Tech. Sgt. Jerome S. Tayborn)

honor and
dignity

you'll know you're a military nurse when …

"…Every day is like an ocean, wave after wave of ill, injured, dying U.S., Canadian, Dutch, Australian, British, Romanian, Polish, Afghan, and Iraqi patients. We care for them all, some to return to their military or civilian life, some to prepare for prison, and some to return home to die surrounded by their families. It gives me peace to know we treat every patient ethically and to the fullest of our abilities."

–Sherri Santos, Navy, NATO Role 3 Multinational Medical Unit, Kandahar, Afghanistan

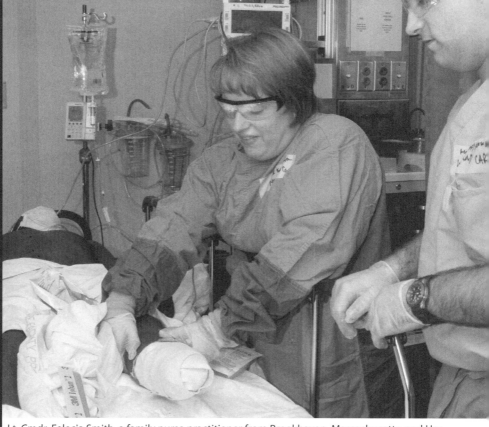

Lt. Cmdr. Felecia Smith, a family nurse practitioner from Brookhaven, Massachusetts, and Hospital Corpsman 2nd Class Steven Buckingham, from Eureka, California, dress the bandage on an amputee patient aboard the Military Sealift Command hospital ship USNS Comfort (T-AH 20). Comfort conducted humanitarian and disaster relief operations as part of Operation Unified Response after a 7.0 magnitude earthquake caused severe damage near Port-au-Prince, Haiti, on 12 January 2010. (U.S. Navy photo/Mass Communication Specialist 2nd Class Shannon Warner)

"…You are dressing the wounds of a man who tried to kill you the week before. As the combat support hospital located with the prison, it was our responsibility to provide medical care to all detainees in theater. Oftentimes, we were subject to attack, as the insurgents were attempting to free their comrades from the prison. If the Quick Reaction Force (QRF) wounded an insurgent during the attack, he was brought to us to stabilize and rehabilitate until he could join the prison population. As members of the U.S. military, we are bound by Chapter 34 of the Geneva Convention, which states that 'healthcare personnel of the Armed Forces of the United States have a responsibility to protect and treat, in the context of a professional treatment relationship and universal principles of medical ethics, all detainees in the custody of the Armed Forces.' When you take care of patients who would rather see you dead, you'll know you're a military nurse."

–*Ann Nayback-Beebe, Army, 115th Combat Support Hospital, Abu Ghraib, Iraq*

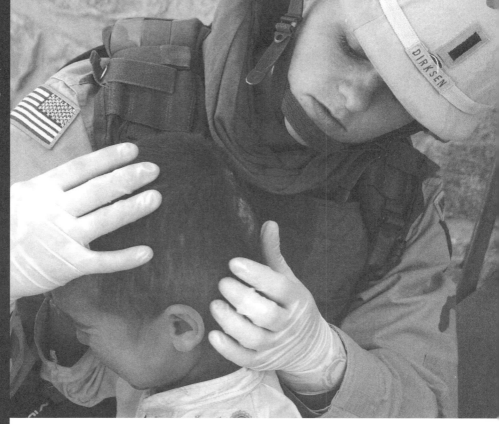

Registered nurse Army 1st Lt. Dawn Dirksen, 911th Forward Surgical Team supporting 10th Mountain Division medical assistance missions in Afghanistan, examines a young girl's head in the village of Loy Karezak, Afghanistan, October 2003. (U.S. Army photo/PFC Gul A. Alisan)

"…You provide expert and compassionate care not only to the soldiers and host nation civilians injured in combat, but also to the enemy lying next to them. He has a devious smirk and scary eyes that you will never forget, but you save his life too and are able to find some approval in that."

–Amber Birkle, Army, Blanchfield Army Community Hospital and 10th Combat Support Hospital, Bassett Army Community Hospital, Baghdad, Iraq

"…You stop for a moment as the lieutenant says, 'She still has nail polish on.' I can only imagine the kind of day the mother had planned for this 4-year-old Iraqi girl. It was supposed to be a festive occasion; one of her relatives was getting married. Surely she could feel the sense of excitement around her, for in these small Iraqi villages, everyone is interconnected. We didn't know whether this marriage was traditional or more contemporary, but doubtless the women of the village took great pride in preparing the bride for her big day. Sadly, sometime during the nuptials, two women dressed in robes released their hatred on the wedding crowd. This happy village event instantly materialized into horror. The little girl, one of 10 injured Iraqis brought to us, sustained significant injuries. Her skin was peppered with black fragments from the blast. We didn't know what happened to her mother.

"As nurses, we can barely absorb the razing of humanity that occurs during war. That is why we only remember our patients as numbers or by their injuries. It is customary that we cannot recall patients' names, and we merely refer to 'the guy with the amputation in bed four.' This is our paltry veil of protection against the brutality that humans inflict on each other.

"That is why the nail polish was so significant; we did not want to see this injured child in front of us, so we blocked out the mental imagery. The nail polish forced us to confront her for who she was. In that moment, we saw our own children and could imagine the caring mother who took time to paint her child's nails for such an occasion. Only when an uncle arrived weeks later did we learn that the girl's mother was killed while shielding her daughter from certain death, leaving the pink nail polish to remind us of how much she was loved."

–Scott Brocious, Air Force, 332nd Expeditionary Medical Group, Balad Air Base, Iraq

"…You discover, above all else, the reverence that the heroes in the combat arms community demonstrate to you. I was involved in some of the worst emergency scenarios imaginable. I saw senior ranking infantry officers and noncommissioned officers break down and thank my young staff for their efforts and 'their tears, because those men were worth it.' It is a picture I will never forget. The most moving and meaningful moment I experienced as a military nurse was when our tour was ending. Leaders from all types of units paid homage to us. We felt that we were just doing our jobs, and they were the heroes who were running the roads with all those IEDs. From the colonel who in the final days could only muster, through choked back tears, 'I will never be able to thank you for what you did for my guys. I just hope you don't take this back home with you,' to the sergeant who, upon hearing what unit I served in, put down his cigarette to shake my hand and tell me, 'Sir, we knew if we got to you, we were going home.' War is a terrible thing, but discovering the brotherhood extended to us from our heroes on the front lines is when you really know you are a military nurse."

–John Groves, Army, Ft. Riley MEDDAC
(Medical and Dental Activity), Baghdad, Iraq

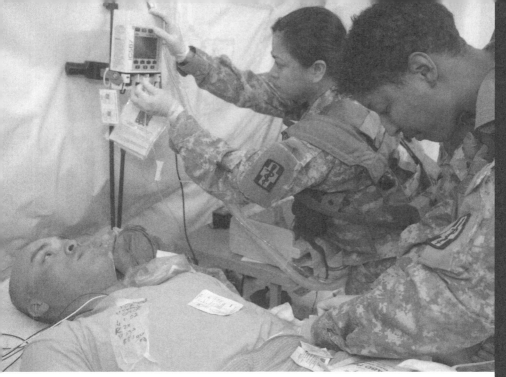

Army 1st Lt. Priscilla Loweright, right, and Spc. Maricris Davison, center, both with the 801st Combat Support Hospital, Fort Sheridan, Illinois, prepare role player Sgt. Robert Demus, a Fort Carson, Colorado, infantryman, for an intravenous during medical training, Joint Readiness Training Center (JRTC), Fort Polk, Louisiana, April 21, 2010.

JRTC integrates U.S. military services, coalition partners and civilian role players into realistic scenarios that reflect current conflicts. During JRTC rotation 10-06, U.S. airmen and soldiers trained alongside Australian and Singapore service members. (U.S. Air Force photo/Staff Sgt. Erica J. Knight)

…You are in the operating room caring for injured coalition soldiers nonstop with triple amputations, double amputations, craniotomies, and so on. Next up is a detainee (the enemy) with a probable fatal gunshot wound to the chest. You watch the team of physicians care for him as if he were a brother or best friend— giving him units of blood and plasma, performing an emergency thoracotomy to keep his heart beating, clamping off his bleeding aorta to send more blood to the heart and brain.

Finally, the decision is made to stop resuscitation. You bring in an interpreter who can guide you in helping this detainee die as he would wish, as the Muslim faith dictates, with the utmost dignity and proper positioning of the head, hands, and feet. You give him the silence, respect, and prayers you hope your enemies would give you in your dying moment, but knowing they probably do not. And then you must move him to the morgue, as an Afghan child involved in an IED blast needs the OR.

–Sherri Santos, Navy, NATO Role 3 Multinational Medical Unit, Kandahar, Afghanistan

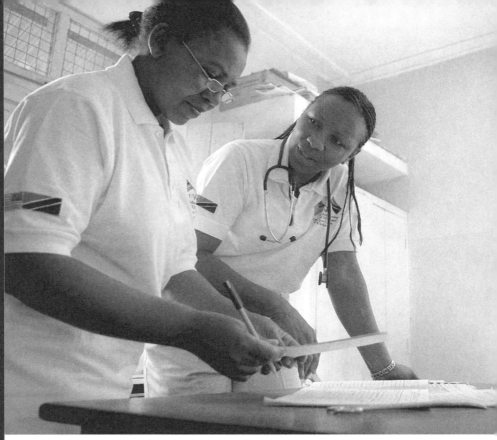

Lt. Cmdr. Lana Cole, right, assigned to the Emergency Medical Facility, Combined Joint Task Force-Horn of Africa, helps a local nurse perform triage at one of the dispensaries during a medical civil action project (MEDCAP) at Tanga Village. Soldiers and sailors worked together to support the MEDCAP in Tanzania. (U.S. Navy photo/Mass Communication Specialist 2nd Class Johansen Laure)

band of
nurses

you'll know you're a military nurse when …

"…You realize that no matter how much you tell your family and friends about your experiences, the only people who truly understand what you have seen and experienced are other military nurses and medical professionals."

–Amber Birkle, Army, Blanchfield Army Community Hospital and 10th Combat Support Hospital, Bassett Army Community Hospital, Baghdad, Iraq

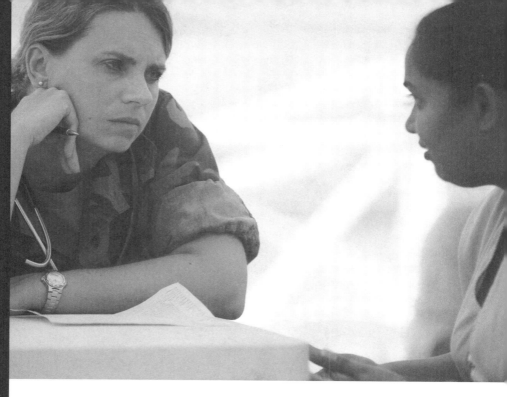

Lt. Cmdr. Kathaleen Sikes, a Navy nurse embarked aboard the amphibious assault ship USS Kearsarge (LHD 3), listens to a young woman during a routine check-up at a medical clinic at the Couva District Health Facility during the humanitarian/civic assistance mission Continuing Promise (CP). Kearsarge is the primary platform for the Caribbean phase of CP, an equal-partnership mission involving the United States, Canada, Netherlands, Brazil, Nicaragua, Colombia, Dominican Republic, Trinidad and Tobago, and Guyana. (U.S. Navy photo/Mass Communication Specialist Seaman Apprentice Joshua Adam Nuzzo)

"…You can't find the right words to explain to anyone what you've just been through. But you are a strong military nurse when you admit you can't deal with it alone anymore, and you reach out and get the help you need. Only then will you know you are an exceptional military nurse."

–*Mary Carlisle, Air Force, 332nd Expeditionary Medical Group, Balad, Iraq*

"…The term 'scope of practice' is an illusion that is 7,000 miles away. When your 'shift' turns into a 72-hour roller-coaster ride that starts in the ER and moves to one medical evacuation flight followed by another, before finally ending up back in the ER. You walk into the trauma bay where you find your battle buddy, who has been covering the ER while you were gone, sleeping in the empty trauma bay. Your buddy wakes up and looks at you, and you both smile, because you know there is no other place in the world you would rather be than saving heroes' lives with the finest individuals you have ever had the privilege of sharing space with."

–*Nicholas Murphy, Army, 115th Combat Support Hospital ER, Baghdad, Iraq*

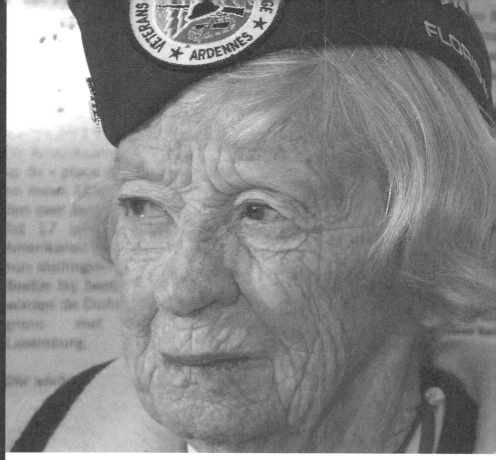

A World War II U.S. Army veteran and nurse who served in the Battle of the Bulge stands and watches as several speeches, presentations, and a 21-gun salute honor the surviving veterans attending the 60th anniversary of the Battle of the Bulge. (U.S. Navy photo/Photographer's Mate 1st Class Ted Banks)

proud to serve

you'll know you're a military nurse when …

"…You witness the pinning of a Purple Heart on an injured service member's hospital gown. He salutes from his bed and says, 'Thank you.' Then, when all the VIPs leave, he says to you, 'This is one medal I never wanted to receive.'"

–Mary Carlisle, Air Force, 332nd Expeditionary Medical Group, Balad, Iraq

…Upon promotion, you wear the lieutenant's bars given to you after the death of a beloved patient, a senior chief who always hoped to one day be an officer and wear the bars given to him by a favorite teacher. He was a proud man who served in the U.S. Navy for the country he loved. He and his devoted wife reared 25 children on an enlisted man's hard-earned salary. He was struck down with pancreatic cancer far too young. He whispered to me that he wanted to die at home, surrounded by his family. The doctors would discharge him only if he could eat enough to get off his hyperalimentation. I ordered him every food that sounded good to him. But he could eat nothing.

One chilly March day, I bundled him up with IVs, tubes, and catheters and took him outside with a bag of peanuts. We fed the squirrels and talked about the changing seasons. A squirrel came up and ate right out of his hand. We laughed and prayed together as the squirrels romped in the grass beside his wheelchair. This breath of fresh air gave him a new determination to get home and enjoy the spring and summer with his family. He struggled, but he did eat when we returned to the ward, just a grapefruit that first meal. Within a few days, he could force down nearly an entire meal.

Soon, he was discharged. I saw the tears of thanks in his eyes. I saluted him and his heroism as he was wheeled off the ward to go home. His family told me he lived to the fullest that spring and summer. He died as the winter took hold that year, surrounded by the ones he loved. They gave me his lieutenant's bars. I proudly wore them later that same winter.

–Susan Lacey/St. Amand, Navy, Portsmouth Naval Medical Center, Portsmouth, VA

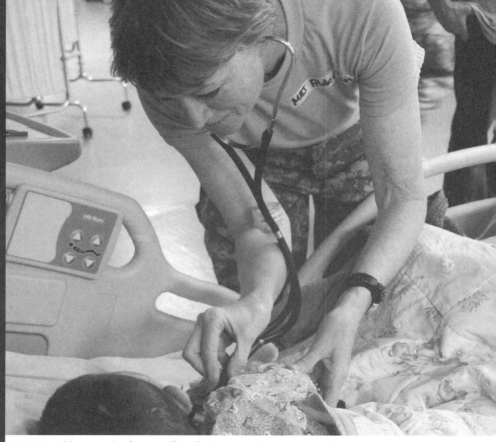

Maj. Una Alderman, chief nurse officer for the 452nd Army Reserve, from Wisconsin, tends to a patient at the hospital on Forward Operating Base Salerno. She was stationed in the same area of operations as her son, Staff Sgt. Seth Alderman, a military policeman. (U.S. Army photo/Pfc. Andrya Hill)

"…You hear Lee Greenwood sing 'I'm Proud to Be an American' or 'God Bless the USA' and get goose bumps. "…You travel abroad and realize the importance of the freedoms that we experience."

–Lisa Lobdell, Air Force, San Antonio, Texas

"…You stand up as the WWII, Korea, Vietnam, and more recent veterans march past you in a parade and realize that you can identify with their sacrifice and service. You recognize that you may have a lot in common, because you too are a veteran of a foreign war."

–Amber Birkle, Army, Blanchfield Army Community Hospital and 10th Combat Support Hospital, Bassett Army Community Hospital, Baghdad, Iraq

"…You work as a team. At first, I felt the community health nurse's job would not be as important in a war zone, but I knew different down the road. I kept my soldiers happy and healthy. During MASCALs, I was the one assigned to the expectants, the wounded soldiers we knew wouldn't make it. Who better than I to hold their hands and comfort them till they passed on?

"I am proud to be a military nurse. I believe I have made a difference in other people's lives. As I look back on my career, I have cared for a lot of patients, but not all of my patients were brave soldiers who would die for their country. I will remember those patients the most, especially the ones who died in my arms."

–*Susan Luz, Army Reserve, 399th Combat Support Hospital Mosul and Al Asad, Iraq*

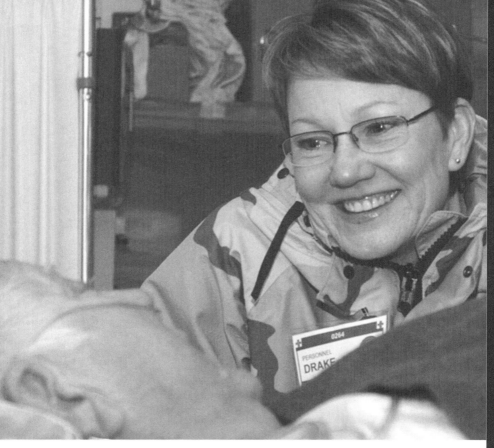

Lt. Col. Beth Drake keeps company with Sam Lee at the Air Force Theater Hospital at Balad Air Base, Iraq, while he waits to be moved to an aircraft. Drake is associate chief nurse of the Contingency Aeromedical Staging Facility; Lee is a labor foreman from a forward operating base (U.S. Air Force photo/Staff Sgt. Robert Wollenberg)

Multitaskers

10. "…You build a 52-bed tent hospital before you start working in it.

9. Every time your patient has to use the toilet, you escort him out to a port-a-potty.

8. Ninety percent of the patients on the ward have a name alert, because everyone is named 'Mohammed.'

7. All the patients' spike temps around 1400 vitals, because it's 90-plus degrees in the tent, and that's with air conditioning.

6. You have mastered the three most important Afghani (Pashtu) words: pain, bathroom, and water.

5. At the end of the day, you walk 100 meters to your tent with your 11 roommates.

4. You are discharging a patient, and you have to know what time the helicopter is landing.

3. On one ward, you are caring for a Marine who has been wounded, and on the other ward, you are caring for the EPW (prisoner) who wounded him.

2. The alert roster consists of, 'Which tent do you live in, and which cot is yours?'

1. Your patient has survived another IED blast and cannot wait to return to his unit outside the wire."

–Megan Dodge, Army, 31st Combat Support Hospital, Camp Dwyer, Afghanistan

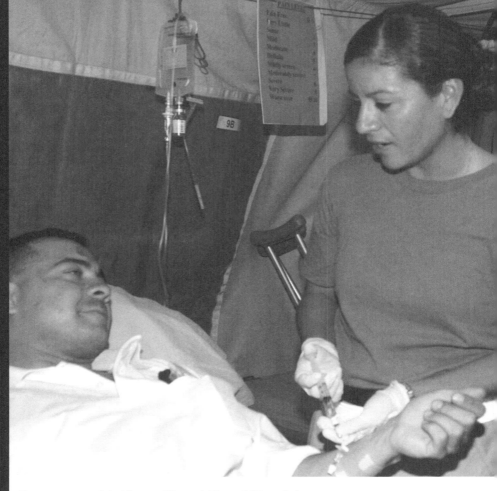

Photo courtesy of the Vietnam Women's Memorial Foundation.

"…You roll out of bed at o'dark-thirty to go for a quick run before duty. You wear combat boots and camouflage to work. On arriving to work, you check the computer and pray your deployed Marine son's name is not on the list of the next medical evacuation flight of incoming wounded from Iraq or Afghanistan. You proudly help off-load litters of wounded and ill patients from the war zone now at the ER door. You quietly answer questions on the phone from an anxious, far-away mother of a wounded soldier who just arrived off a flight from Iraq. You're not surprised to see young soldiers with missing limbs in the hospital. You think nothing of helping a soldier on crutches or in a wheelchair with his or her tray in the cafeteria."

–Lois Borsay, Army, Landstuhl Regional Medical Center, Landstuhl, Germany

"…You're sure they would never need [your specialty]. I was proven wrong my first day. I'm an obstetrics nurse, and I assisted in delivering eight Iraqi babies during my deployment."

–Amber Pocrnich, Army, Ft. Riley Deployed Combat Casualty Research Team/ USA, Medical and Dental Activity, Baghdad, Iraq

"…You write the following: 'I have found myself to be the pharmacist, triage officer, patient tracker, educator, troubleshooter, mentor, coordinator, medical supply and equipment expert, advocate, counselor, peacemaker, confidant, soldier, and above all, the nurse.' "
(Army Nurse Corps newsletter, June/July 2004).

–Jodelle Schroeder, Army, 101st Forward Support Battalion, 1st Brigade, 1st Infantry Division (mechanized), Ar Ramadi, Iraq

"…You find yourself not only in the middle of some dusty, dry country at war but also in New Orleans after Hurricane Katrina and in Haiti after the earthquake."

–Delisa Showers, Air Force, 459th Aeromedical Evacuation Squadron, Balad, Iraq

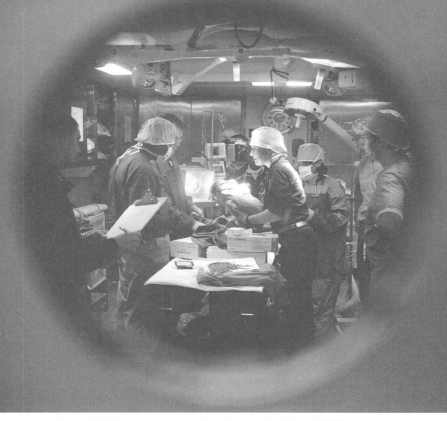

Lt.j.g. Natalie Shaffer, a nurse assigned to Fleet Surgical Team (FST) 8 and embarked aboard the multipurpose amphibious assault ship USS Bataan (LHD 5), hands over a newborn Haitian boy to his father. The child was the first baby ever born aboard Bataan. Bataan supported Operation Unified Response following a 7.0 magnitude earthquake that caused severe damage in Haiti on 12 January 2010. (U.S. Navy photo/Mass Communication Specialist 2nd Class Kristopher Wilson)

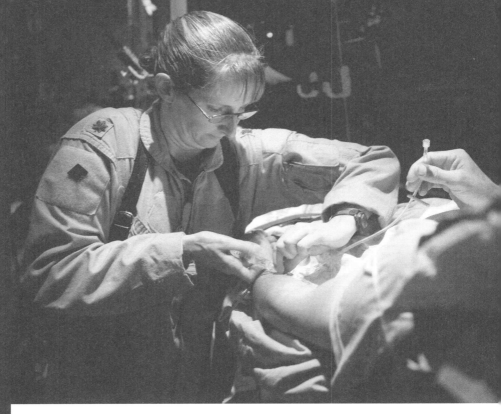

Maj. Missy Steckler provides care to a patient during a flight to a location that can provide a higher level of medical care. Steckler is a flight nurse assigned to the 451st Expeditionary Aeromedical Evacuation Flight at Kandahar Airfield, Afghanistan. (U.S. Air Force photo/Staff Sgt. Shawn Weismiller)

"...You have discovered how much inner strength you have and what you are truly capable of after you finished Airborne School, achieved the Expert Field Medical Badge, completed the Bataan Memorial Death March, or experienced a mass casualty in a Baghdad ER. You learn that you are not only capable, but at your best when you are at the bedside of a casualty playing a key role in the trauma resuscitation and fighting the enemy's attempts to take one more life dedicated to American freedoms."

–Amber Birkle, Army, Blanchfield Army Community Hospital and 10th Combat Support Hospital, Bassett Army Community Hospital, Baghdad, Iraq

"...You hear about nurses stationed in places like Honduras or Africa who encounter awful mud slides, but that doesn't worry them; they will scoop out the mud and keep on cleaning. In the winter, military nurses will overcome snowstorms and drops in temperature. They will not only keep patients warm but also keep an eye on the roof, to prevent the snow from collapsing it."

–Lillian Cardona, Army, 212th Mobile Army Surgical Hospital in Germany

"…Part of your training requires that you learn how to rappel off a platform down a 30-foot wall. … I learned how to land-navigate by map and compass, survive a tear-gas attack, combat-crawl with a stretcher in tow, and operate under extreme duress with the sound of gunfire and bomb blasts blaring in my ears. I discovered that I could do and endure more than I knew was possible. As a military nurse you learn to sacrifice, grow, stretch, and flex, but most of all, you learn how to serve as a part of something much bigger than yourself."

–James Walker, Navy, Portsmouth Naval Medical Center/82nd Medical Brigade, Camp Udari, Kuwait

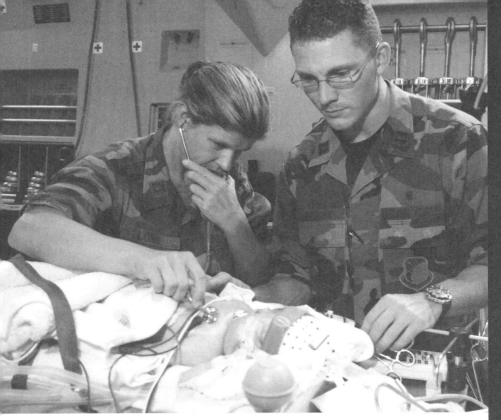

Capts. Karen Long and James Bailey monitor the vital signs and blood flow of 3-day-old Stuart Parker aboard a C-17 Globemaster III. An Extracorporeal Membrane Oxygenation team comprised of Air Force and Army medical specialists from the Wilford Hall Medical Center at Lackland Air Force Base, Texas, flew to San Juan, Puerto Rico, to transport Stuart to San Antonio for more advanced care. Long is a neonatal intensive care nurse and Bailey is a pediatric intensive care nurse assigned to the Wilford Hall Medical Center. (U.S. Air Force photo/Master Sgt. Scott Reed)

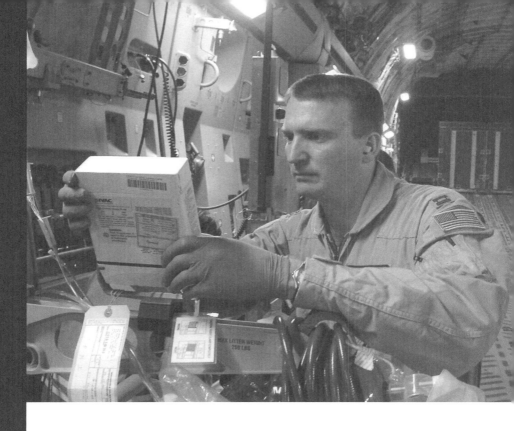

Capt. Paul Simpson fixes an intravenous fluid pump aboard an aerovac mission. In addition to providing patient care, aeromedical evacuation crews must maintain and operate a wide array of medical equipment prior to and throughout each mission. Simpson is a second flight nurse deployed with the 320th Expeditionary Aeromedical Evacuation Squadron/Forward from the 375th Aeromedical Evacuation Squadron at Scott Air Force Base, Illinois. (U.S. Air Force photo)

real life on the
front lines

"…In the middle of the night, you can hear the first crackle of the loudspeaker coming on, telling you 'Bunkers, Bunkers.' When it's all over, you're sure a MASCAL (mass casualty) is breaking down your door, and you aren't in Kansas anymore."

−Susan Luz, Army Reserve, 399th Combat Support Hospital, Mosul and Al Asad, Iraq

María Inéz Ortiz

Capt. María Inés Ortiz was the first American nurse to die in combat since the Vietnam War. She died from injuries sustained during a mortar attack on the Green Zone in Baghdad on 10 July 2007. She was awarded a Bronze Star and Purple Heart, and she was buried with full honors at Arlington National Cemetery.

CPT MARIA INEZ ORTIZ

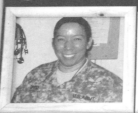 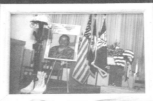 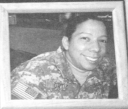

CPT Ortiz was born in Camden, New Jersey in 1967 but was raised in Puerto Rico. She enlisted in the Army Reserves in 1991 and came on active duty in 1993. She earned her Nursing Degree from the University of Puerto Rico and a commission as a Second Lieutenant in 1999. Her past duty stations included Korea, Puerto Rico, and Walter Reed Army Medical Center. She was assigned to Kirk army Health Clinic, Aberdeen Proving Grounds when she was deployed with the 28th Combat Support Hospital in 2006. CPT Ortiz was featured on the HBO series "Baghdad ER" while performing her duties at the Ibn Sina facility. While returning from physical fitness training, CPT Ortiz and two civilians were killed by a mortar round on 10 July 2007. CPT Ortiz was buried in Arlington National Cemetery 9 August 2007. She has the tragic distinction of being the first Army Nurse killed in combat since Vietnam. She is survived by her parents, Jorge Ortiz and Iris Santiago, her twin sister, Maria Luisa Medina, and her fiancée, Juan Casiano. She was remembered for her positive attitude, smile, compassion, and her tireless patient advocacy. A co-worker stated, "IF there was a jewel in the clinic, she was the jewel."

"…You hear that a fellow nurse was killed in action. You pause, reflect, and say to yourself, 'There but for the grace of God go I.' Then you pull it together and get back to work, because your patients need you."

–Mary Carlisle, Air Force, 332nd Expeditionary Medical Group, Balad, Iraq

"…You have emergency plans for your spouse, children, and pets in case of rapid deployment. You save your packing boxes, as you never know where you'll be transferred next. You're tough as nails when it's needed and tearful when you hear a child ask, 'When is Mommy/Daddy coming home?'"

–Lois Borsay, Army, Landstuhl Regional Medical Center, Landstuhl, Germany

"…Showers become available and you comment that 4 minutes is a waste of water, and 3 minutes is plenty of time. We know that in the desert, the sand will always win. No matter how hard we try, the sand keeps creeping in, but military nurses won't let that stop them from daily cleaning."

–Lillian Cardona, Army, 212th Mobile Army Surgical Hospital, Germany

"…You think of the things you see, feel, hear, smell, and taste; the sleep deprivation, noise, and fear (focus). You wonder, *how is my family back home? My dog, my car, my house* (focus)? Here comes another helicopter. *When will it stop? Will my patient stop breathing while I'm taking cover under this desk in my Kevlar vest and helmet? Will she make it to Germany alive? Will his family ever know I was with him as he took his last breath? Will mortar explosions wake me up again?* That bullet hole wasn't there yesterday. (FOCUS!)"

–*Mary Carlisle, Air Force, 332nd Expeditionary Medical Group, Balad, Iraq*

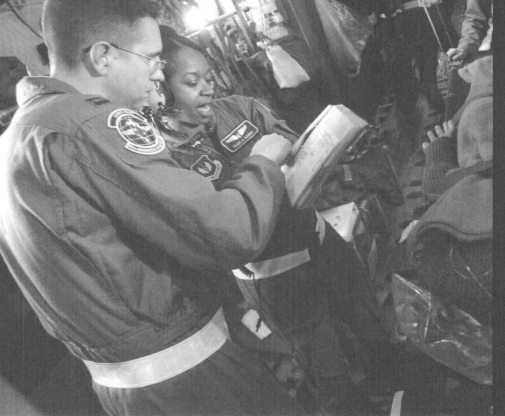

In preparation for an emergency landing training scenario aboard a C-130 Hercules flying over southern Germany, flight nurses Capts. Troy Kinion and Pamela Banks cover a checklist detailing how to properly secure patients and medical equipment for a potentially rough landing. The flight-qualified healthcare providers, assigned to the 86th Aeromedical Evacuation Squadron, fly weekly with Ramstein's 37th and 38th Airlift Squadron's C-130 fleet to remain proficient in their skills. (Department of Defense photo/Master Sgt. Scott Wagers)

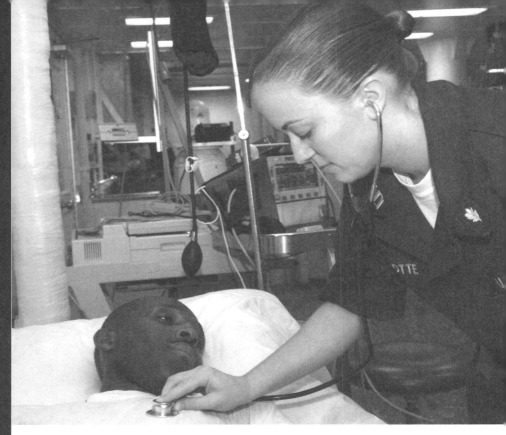

Lt. Ginny Lamotte, intensive care unit nurse for Fleet Surgical Team 8, checks the vital signs of Chief Yeoman Abduel Gibbs for training purposes aboard the multipurpose amphibious assault ship USS Iwo Jima (LHD 7). Iwo Jima is deployed as part of the Iwo Jima Expeditionary Strike Group supporting maritime security operations in the U.S. Navy's 5th Fleet area of responsibility. (U.S. Navy photo/Mass Communication Specialist Seaman Chad R. Erdmann)

rewards of
the job

"…You get to Nellis Air Force Base and think you've landed in 'Top Gun,' and when you feel a pull or an urge to be part of something bigger and better than yourself."

–Lisa Lobdell, Air Force, San Antonio, Texas

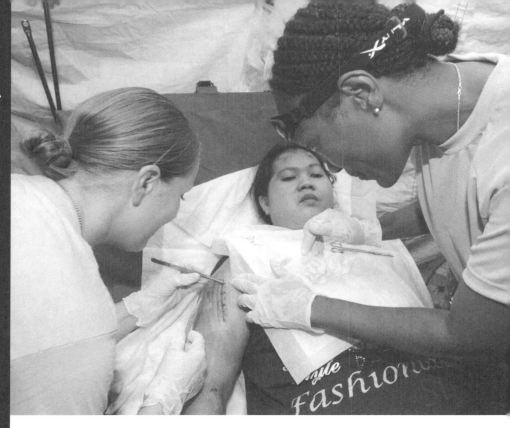

Staff Sgt. Beth Sherman (left) and Maj. Brenda Parker remove sutures in a mobile field hospital in Padang, Indonesia. Sherman, an individual duty medical technician, and Parker, a nurse, were deployed from the 36th Medical Group at Andersen Air Force Base, Guam, as part of an Air Force humanitarian assistance rapid response team. (U.S. Air Force photo/Staff Sgt. Veronica Pierce)

"…Across the trauma bay, the ICU, or the ward, you see 'the look' in the eyes of a fellow military nurse. It is the quiet confidence of experience, of having been tested with the most clinically challenging trauma cases in the world, many of them defying description, and having dealt with them in multiples. And, knowing that you and your colleagues will lean on each other, help each other, and provide each wounded service member the best care possible, not just because they are the most deserving for fighting for their country, but also because they are absolutely the best patients to have—extremely grateful, respectful, and genuinely concerned about their buddies' welfare and getting back to them."

–Joseph Blansfield, Army, 399th Combat Support Hospital, Iraq

"…The reason you, and most of us, do [military nursing] is because of the gratitude we receive from the patients and their friends. Service members know that no matter how badly injured they are, if they reach the 'hospital' alive, the 'docs' will almost always save their lives and return them to their families."

–Terry Mathews, Army, Air Force's 332nd Expeditionary Medical Group, Balad, Iraq

"…At the end of the day, the
tour, the career, you say,
'I'd do it all over again.' "

*–Mary Carlisle, Air Force, 332nd Expeditionary
Medical Group, Balad, Iraq*

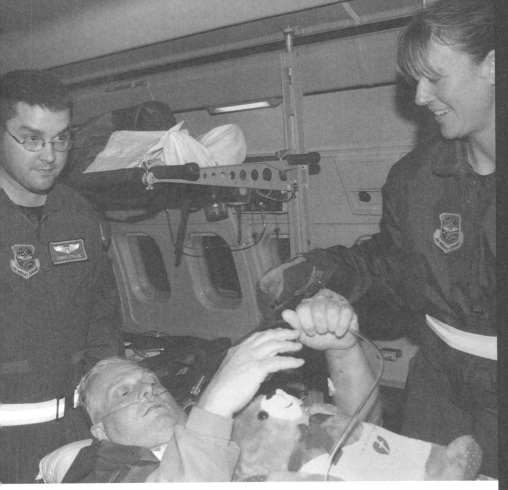

Photo courtesy of the Vietnam Women's Memorial Foundation.

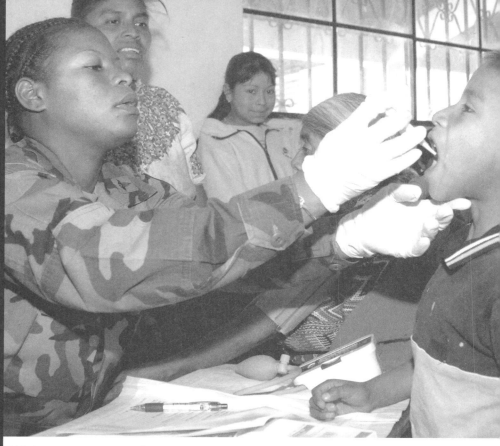

U.S. Army nurse 1st Lt. Arnelle Lewis takes a Guatemalan boy's temperature during a medical readiness training exercise in Santa Cruz Balanya, Guatemala. Lewis is a registered nurse attached to the U.S. Virgin Islands Army National Guard. (Department of Defense photo/Kaye Richey, U.S. Army)

"…You consider it a privilege to leave your family for an extended period of time to perform nursing duties in a Third World country under obscure conditions. I am so proud to have assisted in research performed on our modern-day battlefields. Our predecessors had warned us that we would not be 'just collecting research data,' but in fact, we sometimes would be expected to assist in caring for the traumas coming in."

–Amber Pocrnich, Army, Ft. Riley Deployed Combat Casualty Research Team/ USA, Medical and Dental Activity, Baghdad, Iraq

"…You know it's a heartbreaking honor to fly back to the states on a C-17 sitting next to a flag-draped coffin. You know how to stand and salute when the flag passes by. You're often exhausted and sometimes have nightmares from the things you've seen, but when a civilian or WWII vet smiles at you and says, 'Thank you for your service,' you know it's all worthwhile. You wouldn't want to be anything else but a military nurse."

–Lois Borsay, Army, Landstuhl Regional Medical Center, Landstuhl, Germany

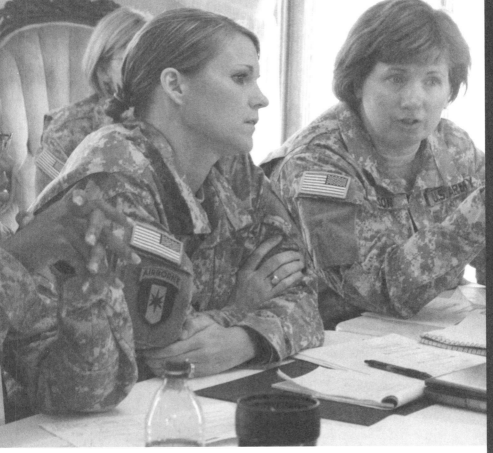

Lt. Col. Kathy Carson (far right), chief of the Clinical Institute for Hospital Education and Staff Development at Womack Army Medical Center at Fort Bragg, North Carolina, makes a point during the Army Nurse Residency program summit at the Stilwell House. (Photo: Jeff Crawley)

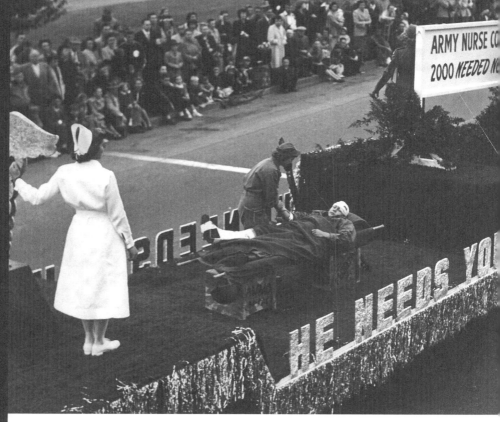

Army nurses 2nd Lt. Betty E. Williams, 1st Lt. Mary I. Couch, 2nd Lt. Donna E. Tolman, and Capt. Alice E. Werner and "patient" Cpl. Harold Collins ride the Army Nurse Corps float in the Armistice Day Parade, Oakland, California, 13 November 1951. (U.S. Army photo/Phyllis [Edholm] Carper Collection, Women In Military Service For America Memorial Foundation, Inc.)

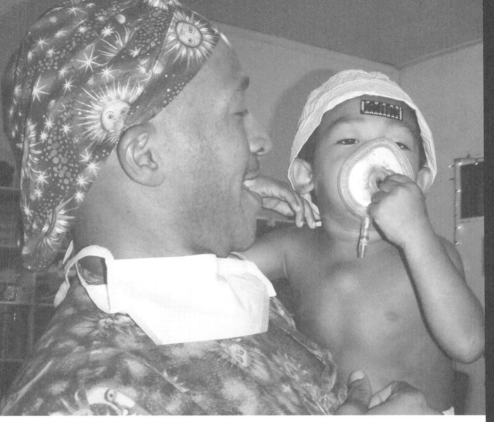

Lt. Col. Arnold Stocker comforts a pediatric patient prior to general anesthesia to remove a cyst on his chest at Jolo, Philippines. Five Air Force medics operated a staffed trauma facility, providing training and emergency and routine care for Joint Special Operations Task Force-Philippines, servicemembers, the armed forces of the Philippines, and occasionally local residents. Stocker is a certified registered nurse anesthetist with Joint Special Operations Task Force-Philippines Forward Surgical Team. (U.S. Air Force photo)

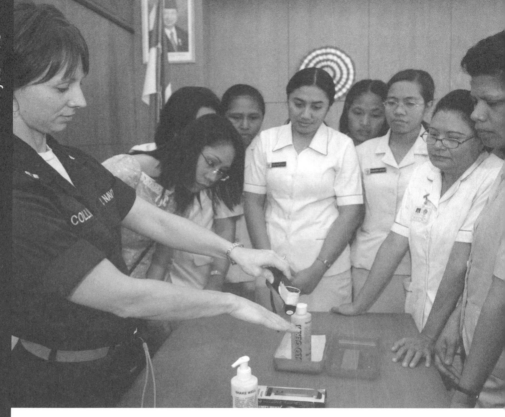

U.S. Navy Lt. Tara Collins of LaGrange, Kentucky, attached to the Medical Treatment Facility aboard the Military Sealift Command hospital ship USNS Mercy (T-AH 19), uses a black light to show germs during a hand washing lecture to nurses from a local hospital. (U.S. Navy photo/Mass Communication Specialist 2nd Class Erika N. Jones)

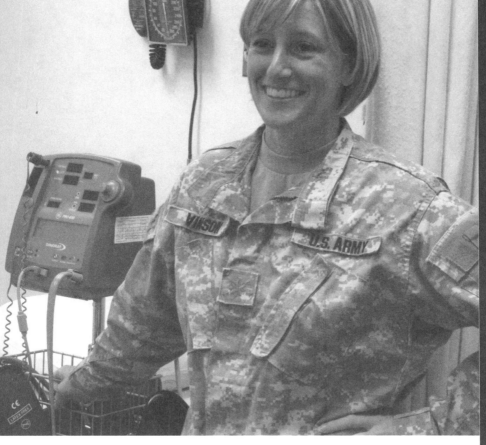

Maj. Elizabeth Vinson, head nurse of the primary care clinics at Fox Army Health Center and commander of the Warrior Transition Unit, said caring for soldiers and their families is a mission that has filled her Army career with once-in-a-lifetime experiences. (Photo: Kari Hawkins, Redstone Rocket Staff)

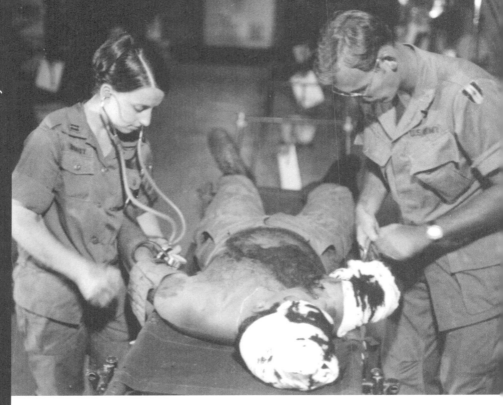

Army nurses Capt. Bernice Scott and Lt. David Van Voohris cut field bandages from a newly arrived patient, 2nd Surgical Hospital, Lai Khe, Vietnam, September 1969.

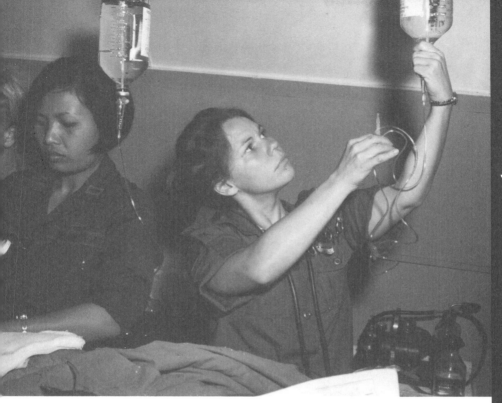

In the 24th Evacuation Hospital emergency room, Army nurse 2nd Lt. Merilee Broushell administers an IV to a patient, Long Binh, Vietnam, 1969. (Army Nurse Corps Collection, Office of Medical History, Office of the Surgeon General)

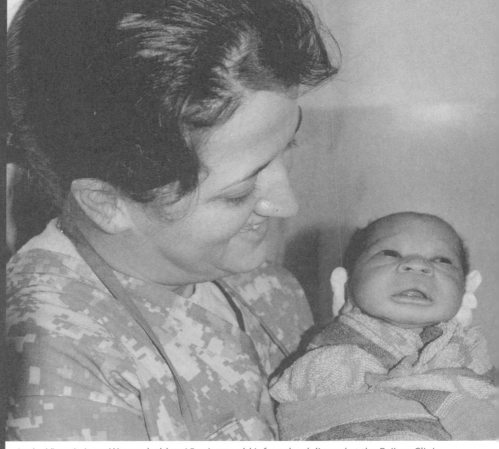

1st Lt. Victoria Lynn Watson holds a 15-minute-old infant she delivered at the Pajimo Clinic in rural Kitgum, Uganda. Watson, an Army Reserve soldier from Abilene, Texas, and deployed with the 7225th Medical Support Unit, is a labor and delivery nurse in her civilian occupation. (Army Reserve Communications photo/Maj. Corey Schultz)

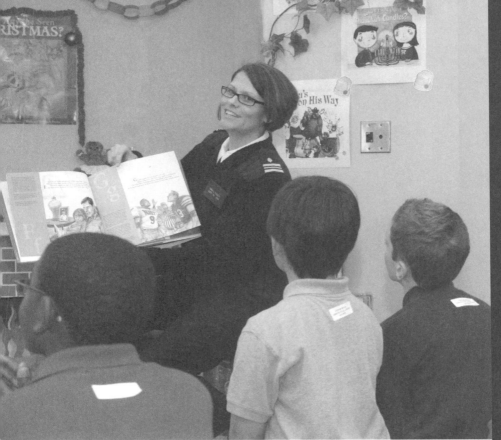

Lt. Cmdr. Sara Pickett, a clinical nurse specialist at Naval Medical Center Portsmouth, reads stories to kids at a bookstore in Virginia Beach, Virginia. The story time is sponsored by the U.S. Marines to help promote its annual Toys for Tots campaign. (U.S. Navy photo/Mass Communication Specialist Seaman Cory Rose)

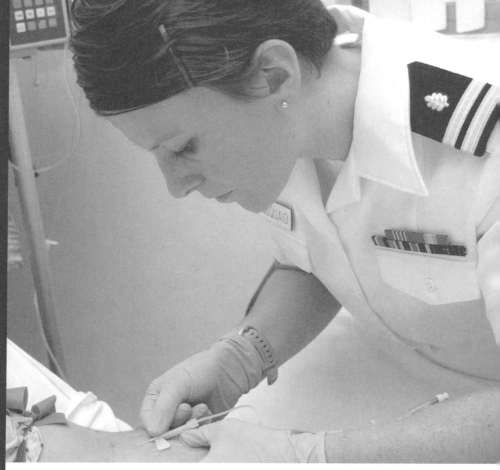

Lt. Erika McQuaid takes a blood sample from a patient who is recovering from a viral infection. McQuaid is a registered nurse assigned to the ICU at U.S. Naval Hospital Guam. (U.S. Navy photo/Photographer's Mate 2nd Class Nathanael T. Miller)

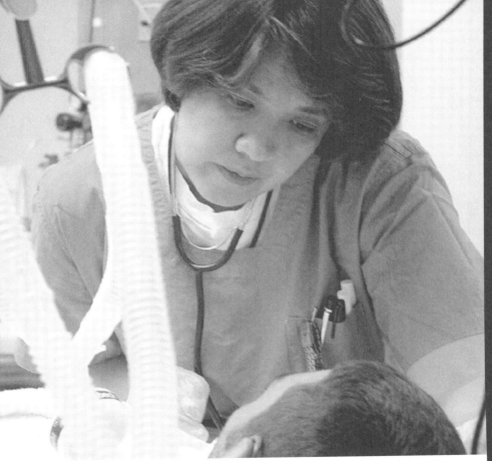

ICU nurse Lt. Cmdr. Mary Ann Brantley, Nurse Corps, works on a patient aboard the Military Sealift Command hospital ship USNS Comfort. Brantley was also deployed in the Gulf region during Operation Desert Storm in 1991. (U.S. Navy photo/Seaman Erica Mater)

Index of Authors

Birkle, Amber 6, 15, 31, 39, 47, 57

Blansfield, Joseph, 69

Borsay, Lois, 11, 53, 63, 74

Braghieri, Tamara, 19

Brocious, Scott, 33

Cardona, Lillian, 12, 57, 63

Carlisle, Mary, 17, 41, 43, 63, 64, 70

Cooper, Christina, 22

Dodge, Megan, 51

Doty, Diane, 9

Dyer, George, 3

Groves, John, 34

Kinsey, Cynthia, 15

Lacey, Susan, 45

Lobdell, Lisa, 47, 67

Luz, Susan, 48, 61

Mathews, Terry, 69

Murphy, Nicholas, 41

Nayback-Beebe, Ann, 29

Ortiz, Michelle, 15

Park, Rachel, 21

Pocrnich, Amber, 53, 73

Quindlen, Paula, 25

Santos, Sherri, 27, 37

Schroeder, Jodelle, 22, 54

Showers, Delisa, 5, 54

Walker, James, 58